POST SEPSIS SYNDROME

Practical PSS Management Guide

Jaylen Fleming

Table of Content

Chapter One

Introduction

After surviving sepsis, a complicated and sometimes misdiagnosed illness known as post-sepsis syndrome (PSS) develops. In this book, we examine doable solutions to deal with the difficulties caused by post-traumatic stress disorder (PSS), providing information on what it is, how common it is, and why having good coping mechanisms is so important.

Survivors of sepsis, a potentially fatal infection-related reaction, develop post-sepsis syndrome (PSS). This illness is characterized by a range of symptoms that are mental, physical, and psychological and persist after the acute phase of sepsis. Post-sepsis syndrome (PSS) is the term for the aftereffects of sepsis that can significantly lower a person's quality of life, whereas sepsis is the body's extreme response to an infection.

Numerous symptoms, such as weariness, emotional distress, cognitive decline, and persistent pain, can be signs of post-stroke syndrome (PSS). These enduring difficulties frequently necessitate long-term care and might have an impact on several facets of everyday living. A comprehensive approach to sepsis recovery emphasizes both the acute medical interventions during sepsis and the continuous care required to improve survivors' well-being. This requires an understanding of and attention to PSS.

Practical measures for managing Post-Sepsis Syndrome (PSS) are of paramount importance due to the persistent and multifaceted nature of the condition. Here's why these practical measures are crucial:

1. **Enhanced Quality of Life:** Empowering people with PSS to deal with continuous issues in an efficient manner improves their quality of life. These steps tackle the various facets of

5

life that are touched by PSS, from everyday responsibilities to long-term planning.

2. **Functional Independence:**Putting into practice practical measures promotes independence by giving people the skills and strategies they need to carry out daily tasks in spite of PSS-imposed restrictions. Self-efficacy and a sense of control are enhanced by this independence.

3. **Symptom Management**: Empirical methods provide concrete remedies for the treatment of particular PSS symptoms, like weariness, chronic pain, and cognitive impairments. This focused treatment can reduce pain and improve general health.

4. **Preventive Focus**: Preventive care is enhanced by practical approaches that integrate lifestyle modifications

and long-term planning. By taking preventative measures, possible problems are lessened and long-term health and recuperation are encouraged.

5. **Emotional Well-being**: By addressing the psychological effects of PSS, coping mechanisms and emotional support given through useful techniques lessen anxiety and sadness. The connection between mental and physical health is acknowledged by this holistic approach.

6. **Sustainable Recovery**: A sustainable recovery journey starts with practical actions. Beyond immediate medical interventions, they equip people with the skills necessary to manage the dynamic character of post-stroke syndrome and adjust to changing conditions.

7. **Patient Empowerment:** Giving people useful advice encourages them to take an active role in their own treatment. Fostering resilience, self-management, and a proactive approach to the challenges presented by PSS require this empowerment.

8. **Reduced Healthcare Burden:** There is a chance that the demand on healthcare services will decrease if people learn to better manage their symptoms and incorporate lifestyle changes. In order to maintain self-care and continuing management, this emphasizes how important it is to empower individuals.

In summary, encouraging a thorough and customized approach to recovery requires effective PSS management strategies. These interventions greatly enhance the overall well-being of people with PSS by addressing symptom management, long-term planning, and the practical aspects of daily life.

Chapter Two

Understanding Post-Sepsis Syndrome

Sepsis is a global health hazard, with an estimated 49 million cases annually. The percentage of people who survive sepsis has increased as a result of aging populations, a rise in chronic illnesses, and resistance to antibiotics; nevertheless, in-hospital survival rates have increased to approximately 80% thanks to recent medical advancements. Consequently, there is a rising incidence of "post-sepsis syndrome" (PSS). Following recovery from sepsis, this illness is characterized by ongoing physical, mental, and cognitive issues. PSS is associated with a reduction in health and life expectancy after hospital discharge, both in the short and long term, and it raises the risk of readmission for survivors.

Causes and Risk factors of post sepsis
- **Biological Factors**

The main cause of post-severe sepsis (PSS) is the body's inflammatory response to a significant infection. Several inflammatory substances are released by the immune system in an attempt to combat the infection. Long-term damage to tissues and organs could result from this excessive and dysregulated reaction.

Sepsis can cause reduced blood flow and inflammation, which can lead to multiple organ dysfunction. The long-lasting impact of this organ failure on their functionality can be the cause of the symptoms that are present in post-stroke syndrome (PSS). The highly stimulated immune system that results from sepsis may cause the immune system to become dysregulated for a long time. This immunological malfunction may be the cause of PSS's long-lasting impacts, which could include an increased inflammatory state or a diminished ability to fight off infections in the future.

- **Environmental Factors**

Sepsis-causing infection severity and duration have a major impact on the development of post-surgical sepsis (PSS). More serious infections are often associated with longer-term effects.
 The timely and efficient delivery of medical care during the acute phase of sepsis can have an impact on the extent of organ damage and the development of post-septic shock. Intervention that is appropriate and timely can decrease the severity of long-term impacts.

Serious infections and PSS may be more common in those who already have health problems, such as immunosuppression or chronic illnesses. Numerous conditions can affect the body's ability to tolerate the stress of sepsis.

There may be an age effect on the body's capacity to fight off infections and recover from sepsis. Genetic predispositions may also have an impact on an individual's susceptibility to developing PSS.

Understanding the development of PSS requires deciphering the intricate connections between biological and environmental components. With the aid of this multifaceted perspective, researchers and medical professionals can create focused therapies and preventative measures to lessen the long-term impact of sepsis on survivors.

Common symptoms and impact

1. Chronic Fatigue: Post-stroke syndrome (PSS) patients typically experience debilitating fatigue that impairs their ability to function and their energy levels.

13

2. Cognitive Impairment: Cognitive symptoms, such as problems with memory, focus, and decision-making, affect overall cognitive performance. It is possible for these symptoms to cause issues in both personal and professional settings.

3. Muscle and Joint Pain: Chronic pain in the muscles and joints is a prominent indicator of post-stroke syndrome (PSS). It can limit movement and create discomfort, making daily tasks more challenging.

4. Sleep Disturbances: The sleep habits of people with PSS are usually disrupted, which makes it hard for them to get asleep, stay asleep, or achieve restorative sleep. This could exacerbate mental health issues and fatigue.

5. Emotional Distress: In PSS, mood swings, anxiety, and depression are typical. The emotional toll that managing chronic diseases and adjusting to a new lifestyle can take is significant for mental health.

6. Functional Impairments: Physical abilities like standing, walking, and holding objects could be hampered by PSS. These functional deficiencies have an influence on independence and daily functioning.

Profound Effects on Daily Life

1. PSS can disrupt professional life, leading to absenteeism, reduced productivity.

2. Individuals may face difficulties in socializing, leading to isolation and potential strain on personal connections.

3. Everyday activities like cooking, cleaning, and personal hygiene can become arduous due to fatigue and physical limitations.

4. PSS can limit participation in recreational activities and hobbies, affecting the overall quality of life.

Emphasizing the Necessity for Targeted Interventions

Recognizing the range of PSS symptoms emphasizes the need for specialized medical treatments. Targeted medications, rehabilitation therapy, and ongoing monitoring are essential for improving overall health and managing specific symptoms.

Including a variety of medical specialists, including physicians, physiotherapists, psychologists, and occupational therapists, ensures a complete approach.

Strategies for physical exercise and appropriate sleep hygiene offer doable ways to lessen the intensity of symptoms. Individuals can overcome the emotional obstacles caused by their illness with the aid of coping strategies like counseling and support groups.

Understanding and managing PSS's complex effects requires educating the public, businesses, and healthcare professionals.

Chapter Three

Medical Interventions

Below are pharmaceutical options aimed at alleviating specific PSS symptoms and improving overall well-being.

1. Pain Management:
   - Nonsteroidal Anti-Inflammatory Drugs (NSAIDs): NSAIDs, such as ibuprofen, may be prescribed to alleviate musculoskeletal pain associated with PSS.

   - Analgesics: Pain relievers, including acetaminophen, can help manage chronic pain and improve overall comfort.

2. Cognitive Function Improvement:
   - Cognitive Enhancers: Medications like donepezil may be considered to address cognitive impairments,

although their effectiveness in PSS is still under investigation.

3. Sleep Disturbance
- Hypnotics: Short-term use of prescription sleep medications may be considered to manage sleep disturbances. However, their use requires careful monitoring to avoid dependency.

4. Anxiety and Depression
- Antidepressants: Selective serotonin reuptake inhibitors (SSRIs) or serotonin-norepinephrine reuptake inhibitors (SNRIs) may be prescribed to address mood disorders associated with PSS.

- Anxiolytic: Medications like benzodiazepines may be considered for short-term relief of severe anxiety. However, their use is carefully

monitored due to the risk of
dependence.

5. Fatigue Management
- Stimulants: In some cases,
  medications like modafinil or
  methylphenidate may be prescribed to
  manage severe fatigue and improve
  alertness.

6. Immunomodulators
- Anti-inflammatory
  Medications:Although research on the
  use of immunomodulating
  medications to treat the chronic
  inflammatory response in PSS is still
  ongoing, it may be worth considering.

7. Symptom-Specific Medications:
- Muscle Relaxants:These may be
  prescribed to alleviate muscle tension
  and spasms associated with
  PSS-related pain.

- Nerve Pain Medications: Drugs like gabapentin or pregabalin may be used to manage neuropathic pain commonly experienced in PSS.

In order to guarantee that pharmaceutical interventions are tailored to each patient's specific circumstances, it is imperative that people with PSS maintain open lines of contact with their healthcare practitioners. Continual monitoring and modifications to the treatment plan can be required in light of the patient's evolving demands and reaction.

Chapter Four

Social Support and Relationships

- Communicating with family and friends: Offer guidance on effectively communicating PSS challenges to loved ones, fostering understanding and support.

1. Choose an Appropriate Time and Setting
2. Be Honest and Transparent
3. Use Clear and Simple Language
4. Share Educational Resources:**
5. Express Your Feelings
6. Use "I" Statements: Frame your communication using "I" statements to express your own experiences and needs.
7. Provide Specific Examples: Concrete examples help loved ones grasp the practical challenges you face.
8. Discuss Limitations and Needs: This helps loved ones understand how they can offer meaningful support.

9. Be Open to Their Reactions: Understand that loved ones may have various reactions, and be open to their feelings and questions. Acknowledging their reactions fosters a supportive environment for ongoing communication.
10.Revisit the Conversation as Needed:**
11.Seek Professional Guidance Together: Involving loved ones in aspects of your healthcare journey fosters shared knowledge and support.
12: Express Gratitude for Their Support:Express gratitude for their willingness to understand and support you.

Effective communication about PSS challenges requires a thoughtful and open approach, creating a foundation for understanding and support from loved ones.

- Educating close ones*: Equip individuals with PSS with resources to educate their support network about the condition, fostering empathy and assistance.

Educational Resources for Communicating PSS to Support Networks:

1. Sepsis and Post-Sepsis Syndrome Brochures: Provides a concise overview of the conditions, symptoms, and potential challenges, facilitating a basic understanding.

2. Online Articles and Websites: Share reputable online articles or direct your support network to reliable websites focused on PSS.

3. Documentary or Video Explanations: Share documentaries or video explanations about sepsis and its aftermath.

5. Books Written by Survivors: Personal narratives provide insights into the journey of recovery and can be emotionally resonant

for both individuals with PSS and their support network.

6. Webinars or Virtual Seminars: Live sessions offer opportunities for interactive learning and Q&A sessions, enhancing understanding.

7. Infographics and Visual Aids: Visual elements can enhance understanding, especially for individuals who may prefer visual learning.

8. Social Media Posts and Articles: Share relevant posts and articles on social media platforms to increase awareness among your network.
9.Awareness Campaigns and Events

Depending on variables including country, geography, sex, education level, and ethnicity, there are significant disparities in the general public's awareness of sepsis. A study employing structured telephone interviews on 6021 respondents in Europe and the US found, for example, that a mean of 88% of respondents in the US, the UK, Italy, France, and Spain had never heard of the word sepsis, compared to 47% in Germany.Of those surveyed, 58% were not aware that sepsis accounted for a significant portion of deaths.

Chapter Five

Practical Tips for Daily Living

- Energy conservation techniques: Provide practical tips for managing energy levels and avoiding exhaustion in daily activities.

1. Prioritize and Plan: Planning ensures that energy is allocated effectively and that important tasks are completed first.

2. Break Tasks into Manageable Steps: This method facilitates progressive advancement without expending excessive energy on tasks and lessens their daunting nature.

3. Time Management: Having a good time management strategy helps you avoid overcommitting and gives you enough time to relax in between tasks.

4. Listen to Your Body:Paying attention to your body's signals lowers the likelihood of

burnout by assisting you in staying within your boundaries.

5. Pace Yourself: Pace your activities throughout the day to prevent exerting yourself too much or too quickly. Maintaining a constant pace helps avoid abrupt exhaustion and keeps energy levels stable.

6. Delegate Tasks: Assign work when you can, asking friends, family, or coworkers for help when needed. By assigning tasks to others, you lessen your overall workload and free up energy for important tasks.

7. Set Realistic Goals: Realistic goals prevent burnout and create a sense of accomplishment.

8. Utilize Energy-Conserving Devices: Make use of ergonomic tools or assistance gadgets, such as rolling carts, to lessen your physical workload.Energy-saving gadgets reduce

physical strain by facilitating more effective work management.

9. Stay Hydrated: Maintain proper hydration by drinking water throughout the day. Dehydration can contribute to fatigue, so staying hydrated is essential for energy levels.

10. Optimize Sleep Quality: Make sleep a priority by setting up a cozy sleeping space and adhering to a regular sleep routine. Restorative sleep is essential for regaining energy and general health..

11. Incorporate Short Rest Breaks: Plan brief rest periods to refuel in between tasks. Short breaks allow for healing throughout the day and help prevent ongoing strain.

12. Practice Stress Management: Include methods for lowering stress, such mindfulness, meditation, or deep breathing.Controlling stress keeps the mind

from becoming tired and helps conserve energy overall.

13. Choose Energizing Foods: Eat foods high in nutrients and energy, like fruits, vegetables, and whole grains. A healthy diet helps you maintain your energy levels all day.

- Planning and organizing for a manageable routine: Guide in creating routines that accommodate PSS-related limitations while maximizing productivity and well-being.

Creating PSS-Friendly Routines:

1. Assess Your Energy Levels
2. Establish a Consistent Sleep Schedule
3. Morning Rituals for Mobility
4. Prioritize Self-Care Activities
5. Break Down Daily Tasks
6. Incorporate Rest Breaks

7. Strategically Place Essential Items
8. Utilize Assistive Devices
9. Meal Planning and Preparation
10. Designate Restful Activities
11. Flexible Workspaces
12. Prioritize Essential Tasks
13. Implement Daily Mindfulness Practices
14. Stay Hydrated Throughout the Day
15. Regular Check-Ins with Healthcare Professionals

Always keep in mind that when developing routines for people with PSS, flexibility is essential. Adjust and adjust routines in response to daily fluctuations in energy and general health. Reevaluate frequently and adapt as necessary to keep productivity and self-care in check.

Chapter Six

Case Studies and Personal Experiences

Real-life examples: Below are compelling case studies illustrating diverse experiences with PSS, providing valuable insights into different journeys of recovery.
Encouraging stories of successful recovery,inspire hope by showcasing stories of resilience and successful recovery, emphasizing that improvement is possible.

- **(Anonymous)** I assumed I had the flu. I was so delusional that I didn't consider calling a doctor or going to urgent care when I started feeling unwell and my temperature went above 104. I reasoned that since it was simply the virus, I would soon recover. By Friday, I was practically unconscious and experiencing strange, bizarre nightmares.

I was texted by a friend, and she became concerned when I didn't reply. She called the police and requested them to come check on me. My house was visited by the police, fire department, and ambulance. Every neighbor was attempting to get me to reply. When I was recovered enough, I opened the door to greet the incredibly polite and understanding policeman. I hopped in the ambulance and headed to the hospital. I was completely delusional about what was happening and was completely out of it.

I had IV antibiotics for three cycles. By Monday, my delusions had terrified me to such an extent that I broke down and went home. (Now that I know why they were so concerned about my returning home.) Despite my weakness and trembling, I was able to take a bath and at last wash my teeth. I received a call from my PCP asking how I was doing and setting up a visit to get checked out.

It required me a few weeks to piece together all that had occurred and make sense of it all. I came to understand that the strange dreams and the events occurring at the hospital were all illusions. Determining what was genuine and what wasn't was causing a lot of mental havoc. Fortunately, my new kidney did not sustain any harm after my kidney transplant, and all of my blood tests came back as normal. Even though I did experience hair loss, I'm incredibly thankful that I avoided suffering further harm. I'll cut a long story short here. The strangest thing that had ever happened to me. Though I do worry that it will happen again,

I've decided to visit urgent care right away if I ever acquire a fever again in order to be checked out.

- **(Margaret Jones)** I had to wear shoes that went all the way through my heel when I was eighteen. After my foot felt uncomfortable for the first twelve hours, I started to get blisters. In the hopes that it will clean the wound, I utilized a foot massager. I started to tremble, scratch, and felt unwell. To get to the ER, I took a bus. By then, I was experiencing a red rash that started at my foot and moved to my ribs. (Infections by Bacteria and Sepsis)

My sister said that I had sepsis. The rash started to go away as soon as I had injections of antibiotics. I was informed that I was very fortunate and that, had I not arrived at the hospital, I might have gone into a coma.

Although I was young and the antibiotics were effective for me, I recovered quickly. I know this isn't always the case, but it's important to never disregard these signals.

- **(Crystal J.)** I'm 39 years old, a dedicated mother of three teenagers, and I balance going to college to further my love of psychology with working a full-time job. However, a history of persistent kidney stones caused an unforeseen detour in my quest. Though they continued to live an apparently regular life, warning flags started to appear. (Kidney stones and sepsis)

I had severe changes in the color and odor of my urine, lethargy, and water retention over the course of three to four months. Due to my hectic schedule, I ignored these symptoms until a crucial event that altered my life's course. I had to call in ill to work because I woke up with terrible kidney pain, which is a common symptom for someone who is prone to chronic kidney stones.

Things became really bad as I bore the agony in the hopes that it would pass quickly. Breathing hard and trembling violently, I knew something was really wrong. I decided to get help right away from a doctor. My ureter had two stuck stones measuring 6.9 mm and 5 mm, which caused a serious blockage, as discovered by a CT scan.

The fight started as soon as the patient was admitted to the hospital and took three excruciating hours to establish an IV. My body began to shut down despite my best efforts, and I begged them to stop. The condition worsened, and I was transported to the intensive care unit (ICU) for emergency surgery as my breathing grew laborious and my lips turned blue.

As the doctors and nurses worked nonstop to stabilize me, the operating table started to fade. In order to combat the infection, they had left the stones in place and inserted a stent before taking out the stones. I discovered that I had been on life support for two weeks when I woke up with a breathing tube in my hands and restrained. The nurse's explanation that my lungs could not function on their own following the implantation of a stent to relieve the obstruction made me realize how serious the situation was. My blood pressure was falling as my heart raced. When both symptoms were present, it could have been lethal.

I struggled mightily to regain control of my breathing once the breathing tube was removed. I took my first breath on my own, gasping but determined. It dawned on me that I had been very close to death. I was unable to walk or carry out daily duties in the hospital as I struggled with the psychological and physical fallout in the weeks that followed. They'd sent me home in a diaper and with a walker. I felt so strong before I got sepsis. In every area of my life, I needed assistance.

Each stride I take toward recovery is evidence of how fleeting life is and how much health should be valued. I'm constantly reminded of my experience with severe septic shock and sepsis, and I'm determined to strengthen myself and embrace a renewed sense of gratitude for life.

- **(Paul Borgman)** This is my story. It started four and a half years ago, at the age of 57.
  Due to non-diabetic neuropathy and stress fractures in my metatarsals bones, I had been battling a chronic ulcer on my left foot. Even though I was receiving frequent podiatric care, my work as an energy engineer required me to walk a lot and conduct field audits, so my injuries weren't fully healed. I started feeling sick a few weeks after going to the hospital for some x-rays on my foot. I had bladder problems, weakness, and appetite loss. After a few days, I began to experience confusion, blurred vision, and incoherent speech. (Infections by Bacteria and Sepsis)

  We went to another hospital's emergency room (ER), where I was quickly sent to a private room because of a clear infection. I was in septic shock, had pneumonia, and my blood pressure was 56/35 due to renal failure. (Septic shock and sepsis, sepsis and pneumonia) My wife was informed by the ER doctor that I wouldn't have survived if we had waited a further 12 hours. I was rushed into surgery after it was discovered that I had an infection in my lower left leg, even though there was surprisingly little seepage from the ulcer on my foot. It took a few days for the tests to be definitive, so we weren't immediately aware that I had an illness like MRSA, as they had suspected. (MRSA with Sepsis)

Thankfully they were able to stabilize my BP and get my kidneys working again.

- **(John Radtke)** I started to show symptoms of illness in mid-September

41

of 2022. My legs and back began to hurt, and I was experiencing excruciating headaches. It progressed over the day and I acquired a high fever with uncontrolled chills. That was a Friday. My left knee locked up by Saturday, and my knees were becoming stiff. Previously, I had both hips and knees replaced. However, at the time, I was unaware that the infection had spread to both knees, consuming three inches of my left femur and causing the replacement to fall apart. By Sunday night, my family had rushed me to the emergency room of a nearby hospital because I was in so much pain and had become so weak. Recuperated Joints and Sepsis

By then, I was starting to experience septic shock. (Sepsis and Septic Shock) My blood pressure plummeted, and I was on the verge of kidney failure when I was moved to a much bigger hospital in Madison. I was in intensive care for the next four weeks, getting both knees replaced, going to dialysis three times a week, experiencing periods of unconsciousness, and having hallucinations.

My lower back vertebrae were infected, causing stiffness and pain that persisted until the end of February when the therapist had me up and walking with the parallel bars, albeit only 20 to 40 feet a day. I was later told that this had resulted in AFIB and that I had suffered a heart attack during surgery. I would spend the next 7 months in skilled nursing facilities, 5 months of which would be spent flat on my back.On excellent days, I could stay upright for little more than an hour or two while using a wheelchair. The medications also produced intestinal problems for me, which led to C-Dif. Like the majority of people in my circumstance, I spent tens of thousands of dollars on medical bills because I exhausted my insurance limits.

I was released at the end of March and placed in a nearby assisted living facility. My body was responding to therapy by then, and I was getting stronger and walking farther with a walker. I was ultimately able to go home by the end of May. October 2023 is now upon us. I still need assistance walking, driving, and working. I've also lost the ability to use three arthritic fingers as a result of this (two on my left and one on my right).It was as awful as it sounds. I began posting weekly updates on my therapeutic progress on a blog back in February. With this and the encouragement of my readers, I've maintained a positive outlook and have kept learning how to modify and adapt so that I may once more reintegrate into the new normal of daily life.

KEY NOTE
Sepsis recovery also differs.To determine a patient's chances of making a full recovery, there are no reliable instruments available. Still, a number of predictive factors have been found. Individuals who have previously been healthy have a better probability of recovering, while those who have underlying disabilities, frailty, or nursing home use have a lower likelihood of regaining functional independence30–35. Crucially, the degree of cognitive deficits experienced soon after being admitted to the hospital does not accurately indicate the severity of subsequent impairments.

With 287 patients and/or family members, 400 interviews were conducted. 70.0% of survivors had completed rehabilitation at six months following sepsis, while 85.0% had applied. solely a small percentage of individuals reported receiving therapy for certain conditions, such as pain, weaning off of mechanical breathing, or cognitive deficiencies brought on by exhaustion, whereas 97% of them solely received physical therapy. In addition to perceiving deficiencies in the timeliness, accessibility, and specificity of therapies as well as in the structural support frameworks and patient education, survivors expressed a moderate level of satisfaction with the appropriateness, scope, and overall outcomes of the offered therapies.

Rehabilitating survivors saw therapy as starting in the hospital, more suited to their individual conditions, and involving improved patient and caregiver education. Both the structural support system and general aftercare need to be strengthened. Less than 25% of treatments deal with conditions including pain, weaning off of artificial ventilation, psychological disorders, or exhaustion. The majority of therapies concentrate on physical difficulties.

Chapter Seven

Conclusion

Many survivors of severe sepsis make a full recovery and resume their regular lives. However, some individuals may sustain irreversible organ damage, particularly those with a history of chronic illnesses. Sepsis can result in kidney failure, necessitating lifelong dialysis, for instance, in a person with pre-existing kidney damage. Individuals with an exceptionally severe case of septic shock may get gangrene that requires the amputation of fingers or toes, or potentially the partial or whole loss of limbs.

Even when they have not encountered the most severe consequences from sepsis, some individuals may nevertheless feel that their long-term health has deteriorated as a result of developing sepsis.

Increasingly, medical professionals are realizing that this is a post-sepsis syndrome, which is the term for the prevalent issues that people with recovered sepsis face.

Long-term consequences and a lower health-related quality of life are common among survivors of sepsis. Sepsis-related impairments in cognitive and/or physical function were reported by 59.3% of elderly US-American survivors of the disease .New diagnoses affected 74.3% of sepsis survivors, and 31.5% became newly dependent on nursing care, according to a review of national health claims data from Germany. Lots of survivors need help with everyday life tasks and are unable to go back to work. There are still few guidelines and effective rehabilitation programs to lessen long-term damage. This is probably part of the reason that a large number of survivors, as indicated by 1,731 respondents from 41 countries in an international survey, expressed unhappiness with the care and support services received after being discharged from the hospital. The World Health Organization and the International Sepsis Forum, therefore, urgently demand that post-sepsis treatment be improved and that dedicated follow-up programs be developed for sepsis survivors.

Rehabilitation programs are one important measure of post-sepsis care. They can help survivors to regain their functional independence.

Made in the USA
Monee, IL
04 November 2024

69310544R00030